The NTM Handbook

The NTM Handbook

A Guide for Patients with Nontuberculous Mycobacterial Infections including MAC

Donita Simpson, M. Ed.

Ginkgo Publishing

This book is not intended to substitute for medical treatment or advice. The reader should seek medical advice from a certified physician in all matters relating to his or her health and particularly in respect to any of the symptoms that may require diagnosis and medical attention.

The NTM Handbook

Copyright © 2005 by Donita Simpson

All rights reserved

LIBRARY OF CONGRESS

Simpson, Donita

For additional copies, please visit our web site at:

http://www.ntmhandbook.com

ISBN: 0-615-36561-2

EAN 13: 9780615365619

Without limiting the rights of copyright reserved above, no part of this publication may be reproduced, stored in or introduced into a retrieval system, or transmitted, in any form or by any means (electronic, mechanical, photocopying, recording or otherwise), without the prior written permission of the copyright owner of this book. The scanning uploading and distribution of this book via the internet or via any other means without the permission of the publisher is illegal and punishable by law. Please purchase only the authorized electronic editions of this and do not participate in or encourage electronic piracy of copyrighted materials.

My deepest gratitude
to my mother,
Genisia,
for her love and guidance.

Acknowlegements

I would like to express my deepest gratitude to Fern Leitman for providing the first and most important information I was able to find about NTM. Her efforts and those of her husband Philip, have most probably saved the lives of many. I would like to thank Mary Allyn of Sarasota, Florida for taking the time to read, appraise and edit *The NTM Handbook*, thank you for your kind and thoughtful efforts. I would also like to thank those at National Jewish Health in Denver who spent hours reviewing these pages; Michael D. Iseman, M. D. for reviewing the handbook and providing his insights; Charles L. Daley, M. D. for spending his valuable time reading, editing and making many valuable suggestions and Lorie Powel, RN, C-ANP for providing her thoughtful feedback. To all the NTM patients that so willingly told their stories and answered questionnaires... your time and effort was so greatly appreciated. Also, I wish to thank Jodi Bollaert for her expertise, support and continued confidence.

*"To wish to be well
is part of becoming well."*

-- Seneca

Contents

Preface 13

Introduction 17

Chapter 1 What is NTM? 19

Chapter 2 Who gets NTM? 25

Chapter 3 How is NTM Contracted? 31

Chapter 4 What are the Symptoms of NTM? 37

Chapter 5 How is NTM Diagnosed? 43

Chapter 6 How is NTM Treated? 49

Chapter 7 Regaining and Maintaining Health 77

Handbook Summary 90

Tools You Can Use 91

Works Referenced 99

Glossary 103

Endnotes 105

Preface

In November 2000, I stretched out on the couch to relax and watch the news. Within seconds I coughed, just one, rather productive cough. I remember thinking that maybe I was coming down with a cold. Later that month, I visited the dentist for my twice yearly cleaning, and as she lowered the chair into a semi reclining position, again I started to cough... gee I thought I was over that. A few days later, I arranged to have a massage to try to relieve some of the everyday tension that comes with any job. As I climbed on the table and laid on my back, the now familiar cough returned, only this time I noticed the unmistakable taste of blood. As the days and weeks passed, almost every time I laid down on my back I would begin to cough and it was almost always accompanied by an unusually nasty taste. When I saw the doctor for my yearly check up, I asked to have a chest x-ray just to be on the safe side. The x-ray was normal.

In December of 2001, I noticed a soreness on the right side of my chest. It was peculiar but feeling quite healthy, I figured I had strained a muscle. Later that month I began to feel kind of feverish and came down with a cold. I did the usual things for the cold but it stayed. On December 24th I saw the doctor and asked to have a chest x-ray because now I was becoming worried. My physician assured me that she hadn't heard anything in my lungs but would be happy to do an x-ray if it would make me feel better. The day after Christmas, she called to let me know that I had pneumonia. After five days on antibiotics, I felt better. The follow-up chest x-ray showed no change, so more antibiotics were prescribed. Since there was still no change after the third chest x-ray, a Computed Tomography (CT) Scan of the chest was done and I was referred to a Pulmonary Specialist. The specialist discovered a condition known as bronchiectasis. Bronchiectasis is a condition that occurs after an infection and leaves the lungs or part of a lung unable to perform their normal function of expelling impurities. Mine was a mild case, and I was probably just having a flare up. A flare up of what, I wondered?

So, now I had a lung condition. I found this slightly alarming since I had always taken care of myself, had never had a serious illness, and no surgeries; I had made it to adulthood without a hitch and was in great health. My symptoms, however, didn't go away. In October of 2002, I decided to see Michael Harbut, M. D. director of The Institute for Occupational and Environmental Medicine in Royal Oak, Michigan. Another CT Scan was performed, only this time, the findings were consistent with Tuberculosis (TB). I was given a TB test and informed that I needed a bronchoscopy and a lung biopsy. A bronchoscopy is a diagnostic procedure where a pulmonologist places a tube, with a tiny camera on the end, through the nose or the mouth into the lungs to examine, photograph and extract tissue or secretions for examination. I suddenly became very apprehensive... What the hell was happening?

The bronchoscopy went well. There was no pain and it was performed on an out-patient basis. After eight weeks of waiting for the cultures to come back, I was told that I had a rare infection of the lung known as Nontuberculous Mycobacteria (NTM). Oh, ok, what are mycobacteria and where did I get it? I was told that I would have to take antibiotics, probably three different antibiotics simultaneously, probably for a period of two years. I was referred to an Infectious Disease Specialist. Oh, my God.

I went home stunned and bewildered but determined to find out whatever I could about this mysterious disease. The Internet enabled me to find articles about mycobacteria but it was all so confusing. I read article after article until I was totally depressed. I learned that the mycobacteria were drug resistant and this was why several antibiotics for long periods of time were necessary.

During my Internet searches I came upon the National Jewish Health (NJH) web site. National Jewish Health offered information online as well as nursing consultants to answer any questions about the disease and treatment. I discovered that National Jewish had a comprehensive program for the treatment of NTM, so with little hesitation I scheduled an appointment and made plans to travel to Denver for an evaluation. The wait for an appointment was three months, and my local physicians agreed that NJH would provide the latest expertise and treatment for my condition. At NJH it was confirmed that I did have a Nontuberculous Mycobacteria known as Mycobacterium Avium Complex (MAC), a form of the disease that would require, in my case, a two-year regimen of very powerful antibiotics (Clarithromycin, Rifabutin and Ethambutol). I would need to begin and continue an exercise program, perform daily nasal washes, greatly increase my protein intake (66 grams daily), and use an airway clearance device that would improve the normal airway clearance performed by the lungs. I was informed that if I did all these things daily and underwent the surgical removal of the middle lobe of my right lung, I would stand the best chance for recovery. I never saw that recommendation coming. What? I thought... I knew the infection was serious, but I had no idea how serious. I listened, learned and tried not to overreact. After five days I returned home to manage a disease that six months earlier I had never known existed.

Today, I am past the initial treatment plan. As of this writing, the infection has improved and I continue to have check-ups every two years as recommended by Charles L. Daley, M. D., Chief of the Mycobacterial and Respiratory Division at National Jewish Health in Denver.

National Jewish Health (NJH) is the nation's leading treatment center for respiratory and immune disorders. The medical communities at NJH are outstanding in the way they interact with their patients. The program is comprehensive, educational, and prepares patients for an extended period of antibiotic therapy and follow-up. Qualified medical personnel deliver instruction and the physician specialists are there to answer questions. I cannot say enough about the care I received and I urge anyone who is diagnosed with this problem to find a way to get to Denver. NTM is a serious illness that can, if untreated, result in death. You owe it to yourself to get the best health care and treatment available; National Jewish will help you get it.

Donita Simpson, November, 2008

Introduction

Who Should Read this Book and Why?

This book provides information to those who may be unknowingly suffering with a potentially dangerous condition known as Nontuberculous Mycobacteria, also known as Nontuberculosis Mycobacteria, (NTM). It is also meant to assist those diagnosed patients, their families and loved ones with information about the disease so they can understand the condition and its treatment.

The Internet makes it easy to find information and research the condition. However, the information is most often written for medical professionals. The layperson is often lost in a maze of confusing medical jargon describing procedures and treatment. This handbook is written to explain, in plain language, what NTM is, how it is diagnosed and how it is best treated. It is not meant in any way to be a substitute for professional medical diagnosis and treatment. If you or someone you know is experiencing the symptoms outlined in this handbook, please seek medical advice.

Why Should You Read this Book?

Human infections due to NTM appear to be on the rise.[1] Michael Iseman, M. D. of National Jewish believes that the increasing number of infections may be a result of some subtle alteration in the ecosystem causing a proliferation of mycobacteria in the water supply.[2] Approximately two people per 100,000 develop NTM infections; data suggests there may be rising numbers of cases in certain parts of the country.[3]

Lung infections caused by NTM, specifically Mycobacteria Avium Complex (MAC), are the focus of this book. With adequate information, those with symptoms may be able to work with their physicians to identify and treat a condition that could otherwise cause organ damage, suffering and even death.

What Will You Learn?

As a result of reading this book, you will be able to:

- Define NTM and recognize its other names
- Discuss predisposing factors
- Identify the symptoms of NTM
- Discuss how NTM is diagnosed
- Describe treatments for NTM
- Find resources about NTM

Chapter 1 What is NTM?

Nontuberculous Mycobacteria (NTM)

Mycobacterium (M.) includes a large genus of bacteria that contain several species. The best-known mycobacteria are *M. tuberculosis* and *M. leprae*, commonly known as Tuberculosis and Leprosy. Mycobacterial species other than *M. tuberculosis* and *M. leprae* are often referred to as Nontuberculous Mycobacteria or NTM. NTM are generally found in our everyday surroundings. They are believed to be contracted from environmental sources rather than infected individuals.

NTM differ from the classic mycobacterium in several ways. They tend to possess:

- A wider temperature range for growth
- Growth rates that tend to be more variable
- Varying patterns of natural drug resistance[4]

In this chapter of The NTM Handbook you will learn what NTM is, why it is important to know about NTM and how you can help yourself to be correctly diagnosed.

As a result of reading this chapter, you will be able to:

- Define NTM
- Identify NTM by its other names and acronyms
- Explain why it is important to become knowledgeable about NTM

> ***Lisa Silverman*** *of Needham, Massachusetts, is 51 years old and has three children. In 2001, Lisa experienced nightsweats but never realized this was a warning. It wasn't until she woke up one night coughing blood that she knew something was wrong. After a bronchoscopy, her sputum cultured Mycobacterium Avium Complex (MAC). She was treated for 18 months with antibiotic therapy. Today, Lisa has been MAC-free for 5 years. She says, "I can be optimistic now. Throughout treatment, I persistently coughed up blood and had many adverse reactions to drugs, but my doctors eventually found drugs that worked. I live as well as I can by exercising, working, and taking care of my three children."*

Nontuberculous Mycobacteria (NTM)

Nontuberculous Mycobacteria (NTM) is a disease of the lungs that can take hold inconspicuously with very harmful effect. It can wreak havoc on your health before you even realize that you are ill. Because NTM infections have only recently begun to be recognized many physicians have not had the opportunity to see or treat patients with NTM. For this reason you will have to either seek out a specialist with expertise in this area or be insistent about having the appropriate diagnostic tests so that correct and timely treatment can be started.

NTM include those mycobacterial species that do not cause tuberculosis, the dreaded and very contagious lung disease that killed so many in the past. MOTT (Mycobacteria Other Than Tuberculosis), AM (Atypical Mycobacteria), and EM (Environmental Mycobacteria) are all synonyms for the same group of mycobacteria. NTM is found everywhere in the environment, for some unknown reason, it causes lung disease in some susceptible individuals. NTM is believed to be contracted from the environment and not from infected humans.

Chapter 1 - What is NTM?

> **Lisa from Massachusetts**
>
> *"I was not as educated about NTM as I am now... I had no other lung conditions and I believed I would be cured one day."*

Mycobacteria

Mycobacteria are rod-shaped bacteria, some of which cause disease in humans. In fact, Mycobacteria like tuberculosis infect more than 33% of the world's population and are the leading cause of death by infectious disease.[5] Infectious disease is disease caused by the actions of a living organism worldwide.[6] The most well known Mycobacteria are M. tuberculosis, the bacillus that causes pulmonary tuberculosis and M. leprae, the organism that causes the skin disorder leprosy.

Often, but not always, people who become infected by NTM are seen under conditions of:

- Immunosupression (the immune system is not working as it should)
- Complications of surgery
- Chronic disease

Human Infecting Mycobacteria

Mycobacteria (M.) most often infecting humans include:

- M. kansasii
- M. chelonae
- M. abscessus
- M. avium complex

Mycobacteria Kansasii

Mycobacterium kansasii cause pulmonary disease similar to tuberculosis. It is relatively easy to treat and can usually be eradicated with only three anti-TB medications for a period of twelve to eighteen months.[7] Unlike other NTM, M. kansasii is not readily found in environmental sources. However, it has been isolated from a small percentage of specimens obtained from water supplies. Drugs that have been successful against M. kanasii include:

- Isoniazid
- Rifampin/Rifabutin
- Ethambutol

Mycobacteria Chelonae

Mycobacterium chelonae is a rapidly growing mycobacteria that causes lung disease. It is difficult or impossible to eradicate, although it has been reported that M. chelone has been susceptible to quinolone (*Quinolones and fluoroquinolones form a group of broad-spectrum antibiotics. They are derived from nalidixic acid*) drugs 20% of the time.

M. chelonae has been found in natural and processed water sources, as well as sewage. M. chelonae is often treated with prolonged antibiotic therapy. Drugs that have activity against M. chelonae include:

- Clarithromycin/Azithromycin
- Ciprofloxacin/Levofloxacin/Moxifloxacin
- Imipenem
- Amikacin

Mycobacteria Abscessus

Mycobacterium abscessus is a bacterium commonly found in the environment. It has been found in water, soil, dust, and animals. People of all ages are at risk. Although healthy people sometimes develop infections with this organism, the disease may be more severe in persons whose immune systems are weak. M. abscessus is one of the most difficult mycobacteria to treat. It is difficult or impossible to eradicate. Four to six medications may be needed and, depending on where the disease is confined, surgery may be indicated.[8] M. abscessus is usually sensitive to:

- Clarithromycin Azithromycin
- Amikacin
- Cefoxitin
- Imipenem

Mycobacteria Avium-Complex

Mycobacterium avium complex (MAC) is the most common cause of infections due to NTM. It is a progressive disease and, if untreated, can be fatal.[9] MAC strains are very drug resistant, although not as difficult as the organisms mentioned above. Some drugs that have been used include:

- Ethambutol
- Rifampin/Rifabutin
- Clairthromycin/Azithromycin

Summary

As a result of reading this chapter, you are now able to:

- Define NTM as:

    An acronym for Nontuberculous Mycobacteria. NTM include those mycobacterial species that do not cause tuberculosis. NTM is found everywhere in the environment, but for some unknown reason, it causes lung disease in some susceptible individuals. NTM is believed to be contracted from the environment and not from infected humans. NTM often infects the lungs.

- Identify NTM by its other names and acronyms including:

    - Mycobacteria Other Than Tuberculosis or MOTT
    - Atypical Mycobacteria or AM
    - Environmental Mycobacteria or EM

- Explain why it is important to become knowledgeable about NTM; for instance:

    It is important to become knowledgeable about NTM so that symptoms of the disorder can be readily identified. Knowing the symptoms and risk factors of the disease can allow symptomatic persons to seek proper diagnosis and treatment if needed.

Chapter 2 Who gets NTM?

Overview

There are many common physical characteristics of people who contract NTM. This chapter of the handbook describes some of the risk factors leading to NTM. It also acquaints you with some underlying lung diseases that could lead to NTM.

As a result of reading this chapter, you will be able to:

- Discuss who gets NTM
- Identify other predisposing risk factors leading to NTM
- Identify common physical characteristics of those who have been infected

---

Mary Ann Werner of Virginia Beach, Virginia, is 76 years old. Mary Ann had been treated periodically for occasional infections but she was not diagnosed with NTM until 2006 when Mycobacterium Abcessus was identified from bronchoscopy cultures.

After eight weeks of intravenous antibiotic treatment Mary Ann felt much better, and regained her weight with good energy. Today, she uses the Acapella, performs saline nasal washes and performs low-impact exercises everyday. As often as possible, she travels to see her grandchildren.

Mary Ann suggests that others with NTM "do as much research as possible about NTM,... get a comprehensive workup at a specialty center like National Jewish Health or University of Texas Health Center at Tyler,... and trust your gut about local physicians... change if you're not satisfied."

Who Gets NTM?

People who are at high risk for NTM infection include individuals with:

- Weakened immune systems
- Underlying lung disease
- Unique physical characteristics (e.g., female, slight build)
- Inherited and/or defective genes

Weakened Immune Systems

Although NTM may result from immunosupression, many people with NTM are not immunosupressed. Immunosupressed refers to the reduced function of the immune system; a state in which the immune system defenses have been suppressed or weakened.

People are said to be immunosuppressed when they experience immune deficiency caused by drugs such as corticosteroids or other immunosuppressant medications. These medications are part of the typical treatment used after organ transplantation to prevent transplant rejection.

Immunosuppression is also a common side-effect of chemotherapy used to treat many types of cancer. Chemotherapy often reduces the number of white blood cells available to fight infection.

Acquired immunodeficiency may be a complication of diseases such as HIV infection and AIDS (acquired immunodeficiency syndrome). Malnutrition, particularly with lack of protein, and many cancers, can cause immunodeficiency.

Chapter 2 - Who Gets NTM?

Underlying Lung Disease

Certain lung disorders may also predispose individuals to NTM by interfering with the normal clearance of mucus from the lungs. When lung disorders exist and/or are excessive, abnormally thick secretions occur, normal clearance can be disrupted. When this happens, mycobacteria can be inhaled and become lodged in the thick mucus, thrive and cause infection. Some examples of underlying lung disease and other predisposing factors are:

Bronchitis

Bronchitis is an inflammation of the bronchi -- the main air passages to the lungs. Acute bronchitis generally follows a viral respiratory infection. The viral infection produces bronchial inflammation, which sets the stage for bronchitis and secondary bacterial infection.

Chronic bronchitis is a long-term condition of excessive bronchial mucus with a productive cough. Chronic bronchitis is also known as chronic obstructive pulmonary disease (COPD).

Bronchiectasis

Bronchiectasis is an abnormal destruction and dilation (widening) of the large airways. Bronchiectasis is one of the chronic obstructive pulmonary diseases (COPDs), defined by the presence of persistent or recurrent airflow limitation. However, the hallmark of bronchiectasis is sputum overproduction.

> **Mary Ann from Virginia**
>
> *"I've known that I have bronchiectasis for 25 years. I've had this closely monitored."*

Cystic Fibrosis

Cystic Fibrosis is a serious genetic disease of excretory glands, affecting lungs and other organs; it causes production of very thick mucus that interferes with normal digestion and breathing.

Emphysema

Emphysema is a condition of the lungs in which the air cells become dilated and lose their elasticity, causing difficulty in breathing. Emphysema is a chronic obstructive pulmonary disease (COPD), which makes the normal clearing of mucus difficult.

History of Tuberculosis

A prior history of lung disease such as Tuberculosis leaves scarring and lung damage that may predispose the patient to further mycobacterial infection.

Inorganic Dust Exposure

Inorganic dust exposure can leave the unsuspecting with a subtle underlying vulnerability to NTM. Prior inhalation of dusts such as silica can render the lungs more susceptible to NTM infection.

Common Physical Characteristics

Research has revealed an association between physical features and vulnerability to pulmonary NTM, more specifically Mycobacterium Avium Complex (MAC). MAC patients seem to have many of the characteristics listed below.

Middle-aged Female

Significant numbers of victims of NTM are middle-aged women.

Slight Build

Smaller, thin women are targets of MAC infection.

Pectus Excavatum

The word pectus refers to the thorax or chest. Excavatum refers to the recessed formation of the breastbone. Pectus Excavatum is a physical anomaly sometimes referred to as "sunken chest".

Scoliosis

Scoliosis is the lateral curvature of the spine. It is a common anomaly and can range in severity from slight to severe.

Mitral Valve Prolapse

This is a condition of the Mitral Valve of the heart. It refers to the back flow of blood through the valve ranging in severity from slight to severe.

Inherited and Defective Genes

Studies at National Jewish Health reveal that many NTM patients are genetically predisposed to lung infections. Many have inherited one of the genes for Cystic Fibrosis while others have a defective alpha-1 anti-trypsin gene (a condition that has been connected to emphysema).

When a person with a predisposing condition like the gene for Cystic Fibrosis is exposed to aerosolized water containing mycobacteria, they may be the perfect candidates for NTM. (Water becomes aerosolized when ultramicroscopic particles are dispersed or suspended in air or gas. We may be exposed to aerosolized water in an indoor pool or hot tub, fountain or shower.)

Summary

As a result of reading this chapter, you are now able to:

- Discuss who gets NTM, for instance those with:
  - Weakened immune systems
  - Inherited and/or genetic defects
- Identify other predisposing risk factors for NTM, for example:
  - Emphysema
  - History of tuberculosis
  - Bronchiectasis
  - Cystic fibrosis
  - Chronic bronchitis due to cigarette smoking
  - Inorganic dust exposure
- Identify some of the physical characteristics of those who have been infected with NTM, for instance:
  - Middle-aged females
  - Slightly built women
  - Pectus Excavatum
  - Scoliosis
  - Mitral Valve Prolapse

Chapter 3   How is NTM Contracted?

Overview

This chapter will explain how NTM is most likely contracted.

As a result of reading this chapter you will be able to:

- Discuss the sources of NTM
- Identify some reasons for susceptibility of infection
- Explain how NTM might be contracted

> **Nancy Soucy**, 51 years old, lives in Florida where the largest numbers of NTM patients reside. She says..."It all started with a strange pain in my upper right chest. My primary care physician diagnosed pleurisy and sent me for a chest x-ray. Pneumonia was diagnosed and I was put on a Z-Pack (Azithromycin), for 10 days. Meanwhile the pain disappeared. Weeks later I was sent for a second chest x-ray which revealed no improvement. Another course of antibiotics; this time Biaxin was prescribed. Weeks later there was no improvement. My primary care physician sent me to a pulmonologist who suspected MAC right away. He had a handful of NTM patients in his 20+ years of practice. He did a bronchoscopy and the culture came back positive for MAC. He started me on antibiotics that were commonly prescribed for MAC: Biaxin, Ethanbutol and Rifampin. I also had pulmonary function tests; commonly called PFTs which were within normal range.

Nancy from Florida, continued

After some time on the drugs I was not feeling much better. I was tired, short of breath and coughing. I decided to go to National Jewish Health for their two week evaluation program. Almost one year from the start of my problem, I was admitted to NJ.

Well, I was in for a shock! At National Jewish, I was found to have M. Avium (MAC), M. Abscessus, Pseudomona Aeruginosa and bronchiectasis. I was started on Intravenouis Primaxin and Inhaled Amikacin, along with an Atrovent inhaler. These three antibiotics were added to my original three drugs. I am now taking six drugs on a daily basis. I had a PICC (peripherally inserted central catheter) line put in. They taught me how to use the Acapella, an airway clearance device. I was released and back in Florida I had a home health care nurse come in once a week to change my PICC line and bandage. I was taught to give myself the IV with no problem.

Six months later I returned to Denver for reevaluation; since there was not much improvement, surgery of the left lung was recommended. I was hesitant. I told them I would think about it. Meanwhile I heard of a study at NIH for MAC patients; I applied and was accepted. On my first visit, I asked them if they felt I would benefit from surgery. They agreed with NJH so, I had the surgery a month later in Denver. In two weeks I was home and fully recovered in two months. A few months later I started my first "drug holiday".

Several months later, a CT scan revealed worsening in right lung. A bronchoscopy revealed that I had Serratia, a new bacterium for me. Cipro was prescribed for three weeks seemed to clear that up. Several months later, I had pleurisy in right lung on several occasions. After a follow-up visit to NIH, I was told that I had new infections in my right lung. When I returned home to Florida...

Nancy from Florida, continued

I had another bronchoscopy. I know that I face possible surgery again in the future.

From the start of this story to now, it's been 4 years of tests, treatments, traveling to hospitals, etc. This disease is very complicated and treatment is cautious at best. Hopes for remission remain, but in my case, just when I think I am getting better, a new infection occurs. I will continue to visit the best hospitals, for me these are NIH in Bethesda, Maryland and National Jewish Health in Denver. I am grateful to have a local pulmonologist who cares and is trying to help me.

In my day to day life, I thank God for allowing me to continue to be an active person. I play golf several days a week, but I have to ride in a golf cart. I work out at a local gym when I can, or walk. Living in Florida allows me these activities year round. I am involved with my church and I consider myself a spiritual person. Friends have rallied around me with support and love. The love of my family cushions the hurt and frustrations of this disease. I believe God has a purpose for my life, and this illness is part of the journey to fulfill this purpose. We can never give up hope, seeking answers as much as we can, participating in treatments whenever available. Think about contributing to the future by enlisting in the study programs offered at NIH or other places. Talk to people whenever an opportunity arises about this disease.

But I think the most important thing is to keep a smile on your face and a positive attitude toward it all. Do ask for help, but do not expect it. It is up to us to help ourselves through education, research, prayer and hope. I pray that my story helps others going through this. God Bless us all."

Sources of NTM

NTM are bacteria generally found in water and soil; they are everywhere in the environment. They are contracted from environmental sources rather than infected humans.

Aerosolized water is currently believed to be the most likely source of infection. Human-to-human or animal-to-human transmission is rare. NTM infections do seem to have some geographic concentrations. Mycobacterium avium-complex is commonly seen in southeast parts of the United States, whereas M. kansasii is more common in the Midwest. The initial site of entry is probably the lung.

Susceptibility of Infection

Individuals susceptible to NTM, as mentioned in Chapter 2, are those with certain predisposing conditions, such as:

- Weakened immune systems
- Underlying lung disease
- Anatomical defects
- Inherited or defective genes

In addition, research suggests that inorganic dust exposure can also be a precursor to contracting NTM. Inorganic dust is airborne particulate matter from inorganic sources like silica, asbestos, iron, mercury, etc.

How NTM May Be Contracted

Mycobacteria are everywhere in the environment. They are found in soil and water. They flourish in the biofilms of ponds, lakes and water reservoirs; they are even known to grow inside the faucets and pipes of household plumbing. Water that would normally be harmless may become hazardous to those who are susceptible. NTM may be contracted when the fine mist of a shower, hot tub, or heated indoor swimming pool containing mycobacteria is breathed deep into the lungs. As of 2008 data coming from the Virginia

Tech RIPS Water Study supports the hypothesis that household water systems are a source of NTM infection.

NTM Cases Increasing

It is unclear why NTM infections seem to be increasing at a significant rate in North America. Increases of NTM (MAC specifically), which began before the onset of AIDS in this country, are not due to the HIV impact on the population. The current increase in NTM cases include:

- Individuals who do not have predisposing lung disease
- A disproportionate number of women
- More cases of young people

Nancy from Florida

"We worry yes, so allow yourself to worry for an hour, then move on. Life is too short to spend it on useless stuff, whether you are sick or not. Don't you agree?"

Summary

As a result of reading this chapter you will be able to:

- Discuss the origins of NTM, for instance:
  - It is believed that NTM is everywhere in the environment, and is contracted from environmental sources rather than infected humans

- Explain how NTM might be contracted, for example breathing the warm mist from:
  - Showers
  - Hot tubs

- Identify some reasons for susceptibility of infection, for instance individuals with:
  - Weakened immune systems
  - Underlying lung disease
  - Predisposing anatomical defects
  - Inherited genes and or defective genes
  - Previous inorganic dust exposure

Chapter 4 What are the Symptoms of NTM?

Overview

Recognizing the symptoms of NTM and consulting with a pulmonary specialist in a timely manner are critical steps in the diagnosis and treatment of NTM. In this chapter you will become familiar with the symptoms of NTM infection.

As a result of reading this chapter, you will be able to:

- Recognize the symptoms of NTM infection
- Identify specific characteristics of those symptoms
- Decide when to see your physician

> **Sandy Solomon,** *a 68 year old clinical audiologist from Armonk, New York, is married and has three sons, David, Andrew and Jeffery. Sandy and her husband Alan are both retired and they have two granddaughters. Sandy first experienced the gradual onset of a cough when she was 57. Her Ear, Nose and Throat (ENT) specialist treated her for bronchitis but when her cough persisted and night sweats occurred she saw an infectious disease specialist who did a routine TB test. Sandy was diagnosed and treated for Tuberculosis. After two weeks of treatment Sandy displayed an allergic reaction to the medication which forced a visit to a TB specialist in Newark, he confirmed that Sandy did not have TB but NTM. After several medications were added to the drug regimen Sandy became ill and frustrated.*

> **Sandy from New York, continued**
>
> *Several specialists later, Sandy was finally referred to National Jewish Health in Denver; there she was put on three powerful antibiotics for the treatment of a mycobacterial infection known as Mycobacterium Avium Complex (MAC).*
>
> *Sandy finished her initial drug therapy after 2½ years but relapsed after 4 years without drugs. Today, Sandy continues treatment but insists that SHE controls the disease… and that it does not control her. She is active with NTMir (Nontuberculous Mycobacteria Information and Research) and goes to Washington to lobby congress for funds to conduct much needed research for this disease.*

Symptoms

Overall, the symptoms of pulmonary mycobacterial infections, including MAC, are the same. They may include:

- Chronic cough
- Sputum production
- Weight loss
- Shortness of breath
- Fatigue
- Chest pain
- Hemoptysis (bloody sputum)
- Low-grade fever
- Nightsweats

Chronic Cough

A chronic cough is one that doesn't seem to go away. Many of those diagnosed with NTM complain of an unusual chronic cough. For some, the cough is only demonstrated while in a reclining position. The cough persists and usually produces a disagreeable taste. Occasionally, the sputum produced contains blood.

> **Sandy from New York**
>
> *"My story begins in the fall of 1993, at the age of 54, with the gradual onset of a cough which was diagnosed as "allergic bronchitis". My cough increased, I had night sweats and in February of 1994, I consulted an infectious disease specialist."*

Sputum Production

Sputum is the material that is produced from the lungs. In normal lungs, sputum is often produced during a cough. Even when a cough is present, sputum can be difficult to expectorate (cough out).

Hemoptysis

Hemoptysis is the coughing of blood from the lungs or bronchial tubes. Some patients complain of spitting up blood or finding blood in the sputum produced by a cough. Some patients, who find it difficult to cough, or find it impossible to produce any sputum even if they do cough, often mention that they sometimes detected the taste of blood while coughing.

Weight Loss

Weight loss and loss of appetite are symptoms that often accompany NTM. Many NTM patients complain that they have no appetite and were unable to eat in a normal fashion for some time preceding diagnosis.

Shortness of Breath

Breathlessness has also been a frequent complaint from those diagnosed with NTM. The most normal activity would leave some patients out of breath. Often walking just short distances would labor the breathing of those with NTM.

Fatigue

NTM patients often complain of unusual fatigue. When activities that normally cause little or no fatigue begin to slow you down or make you question what is happening, seek medical advice.

Chest Pain

Chest pain is a common complaint of NTM patients. Chest pain should never be ignored; see your physician or get to an emergency room as soon as possible.

Low Grade Fever

Normal body temperature varies among people; the average is 98.6°F. Body temperatures from 99°F to 100°F are considered low-grade fevers. Anything over 100°F is classified as a fever. Many NTM patients have mentioned that they experienced low-grade fevers but, because they were low, they were often ignored.

Night Sweats

Night sweats are the profuse sweating at night occurring in the course of pulmonary tuberculosis and other debilitating diseases. Night sweats are also a symptom of menopause. For women of middle age this symptom, coupled with any other symptoms of NTM, must be taken very seriously.

See a Doctor

A chronic, persistent cough is enough reason to see a doctor. Chronic cough coupled with any of the previously mentioned symptoms warrants a conversation with a physician specializing in pulmonary medicine or infectious disease.

NTM is a serious infectious disease. Anyone experiencing symptoms of NTM should immediately seek out the best specialists and treatment available.

Sandy from New York

"I consulted several physicians, both pulmonologists and infectious disease specialists in New York City; each was unsure of the appropriate treatment and recommended that I go to National Jewish Health in Denver."

Summary

As a result of reading this chapter, you are now able to:

- Recognize the symptoms of NTM infection including:
    - Chronic cough
    - Sputum production
    - Weight loss
    - Shortness of breath
    - Fatigue
    - Chest pain
    - Hemoptysis
    - Low-grade fever
    - Nightsweats

- Identify specific characteristics of symptoms such as:
    - Chronic cough often demonstrated while reclining
    - Sputum production with blood
    - Nightsweats that wake one from sleep with perfuse sweating
    - Unexplained, persistent fevers above normal (98.6° but below 100°F)

- Recognize that it's time to see a doctor when:
    - Chronic cough is accompanied by fatigue, chest pain and nightsweats
    - Chest pain is present
    - Coughing blood
    - Low grade fever, weight loss and fatigue are troubling

Chapter 5 How is NTM Diagnosed?

Overview

Once symptoms have been observed, correct and quick diagnosis is essential for resolution of symptoms and cure. In this chapter you will become acquainted with the way in which NTM is diagnosed and the diagnostic procedures that are necessary to correctly identify the condition. You will also learn why correct diagnosis is so important.

As a result of reading this chapter you will be able to:

- Identify the necessary procedures for diagnosis of NTM
- Discuss why correct diagnosis is so important

***Deanna York** of Tyler, Texas is a 61 year old Registered Nurse. She was officially diagnosed with NTM in April of 2001 and in October of 2004 she was referred to University of Texas Health Center in Tyler Texas where she received specialty treatment for NTM. Her sputum samples have been negative since 2006.*

Today, Deanna maintains her current state of health by exercising three to four times a week, using both cardio and weight training and maintaining a healthy diet. She also keeps a positive attitude, receives support and encouragement from others, and gets lots of rest.

Deanna encourages those with NTM to: "consider meeting your own needs first, before attempting to deal with all the expectations of society, family and work, this is quite important for those of us who have pulmonary disease (or any other chronic disease)."

Diagnostic Procedures

Typical diagnostic procedures necessary for the discovery of NTM include:

- Medical history and symptoms
- Chest X-Ray (CXR)
- Pulmonary function test (PTF)
- Computed Tomography (CT) scan of the chest
- Sputum culture
- Bronchoscopy

Medical History and Symptoms

Your medical history is the recording of illnesses, surgeries and conditions for further review. Your physician will need to know the medical history of your immediate family as well. Knowing which illnesses you and your family have had will provide your doctor with a picture of any underlying lung conditions.

Understanding current symptoms will help your doctor get a complete picture of what may be happening to your health.

Chest X-Ray

The chest x-ray is an x-ray of the chest cavity, lungs, heart, large arteries, ribs and the diaphragm. The test is performed in a hospital radiology department or in the health care provider's office by an x-ray technician. Two views are usually taken; one in which the x-rays pass through the chest from back to front (posterior-anterior view) and the other in which the x-rays pass through the chest from one side to the other (lateral view).

Chapter 5 - How is NTM Diagnosed?

Pulmonary Function Test

Pulmonary function tests are a broad range of tests that are usually done in a health care provider's office or a specialized facility. They measure how well the lungs take in and exhale air, and how efficiently they transfer oxygen into the blood.

CT Scan

A computed tomography (CT) scan is a method of body imaging in which a thin x-ray beam rotates around the patient.

A computer analyzes the data to construct a cross-sectional image. These images can be stored, viewed on a monitor, or printed on film. In addition, three-dimensional models of organs can be created by stacking the individual images or "slices."

Sputum Culture

Sputum is the substance that comes up with deep coughing; it is a secretion produced in the lungs and the bronchi (tubes that carry the air to the lung). This mucus-like secretion may become infected, bloodstained, or contain abnormal cells that may lead to a diagnosis.

Sputum samples are collected by coughing up liquid from the lungs. The sputum is then taken to the laboratory where it is placed in a medium under conditions that allow any foreign or invading organisms to grow. These cultures are then tested to help identify the bacteria that are causing infection in the lungs or the airways (bronchi). Sputum cultures can take several weeks to complete.

Bronchoscopy

A bronchoscopy is a diagnostic procedure in which a tube with a tiny camera on the end is inserted through the nose or mouth into the lungs. The procedure provides a view of the lungs/airways and allows doctors to collect lung secretions and biopsy tissue specimens. A bronchoscopy is recommended if a chest x-ray or other diagnostic procedure suggests a lung disease that requires closer inspection of the airways and/or the lung. A biopsy -- the removal of a small piece of tissue for microscopic examination and/or culture -- often helps the physician make a diagnosis.

Bronchoscopy is also recommended if you have been coughing up blood (hemoptysis).

> **Deanna from Texas**
>
> *"A chest x-ray revealed unusual scarring and adhesions. A bronchoscopy later that year produced washings that grew MAI (Mycobacterium Avium Intracellulare)."*

Correct Diagnosis

NTM infections are difficult to diagnose. If NTM is suspected it is important to identify the type of mycobacteria, so that appropriate treatment can be administered. Some people with NTM appear to remain well, while others develop serious progressive disease.

It is becoming evident that NTM is a condition that is probably not rare. It is, however frequently misdiagnosed. A pulmonary or infectious disease specialist is probably your first step in correctly diagnosing and treating NTM. The treatment of NTM is complex and lengthy; therefore it is prudent to have a specialized lab analyze your sputum or tissues.

Summary

As a result of reading this chapter, you are now able to:

- Identify typical diagnostic procedures necessary for the discovery of NTM including:
    - Medical history and symptoms
    - Chest X-Ray (CXR)
    - Pulmonary Function Test (PTF)
    - Computed Tomography (CT) scan of the chest
    - Sputum Culture
    - Bronchoscopy
- Discuss why correct diagnosis is so important; for instance:
    - Because NTM is a serious disease that can cause serious progressive disease it is important to receive proper diagnosis and treatment.
    - Since mycobacteria are drug resistant it is most important to identify and treat the exact organism.

Chapter 6   How is NTM Treated?

Overview

In this chapter, you will be introduced to some of the major antibiotics used to treat NTM. These explanations are not a substitute for professional medical advice. This discussion is provided for NTM patients who may already be using the identified antibiotics to point out allergic and or adverse reactions.

As a result of reading this chapter you will be able to:

- Identify typical treatments for NTM
- Identify some of the major antibiotics used to treat NTM
- Discuss other things you might do to help improve your rate of recovery and health

Carole LaMontagne of Hamilton, Massachusetts, is 65 years old. She has experienced several bouts of pneumonia since 1973. From 1984-1994 Carole experienced severe chest pain, shortness of breath, fatigue, chronic cough and low grade fever. It wasn't until 2002 when Carole visited National Jewish Health in Denver that she was correctly diagnosed. By this time, Carole had advanced stages of MAC in both lungs and was advised to have surgery to remove her right middle lobe. In 2003, surgery was performed; Carole now takes oral medication seven days a week and IV antibiotics five days a week.

Today, Carole keeps a positive attitude and takes an active role in maintaining her health; she makes it a point to keep stress to a minimum. Carole suggests that those with NTM "be active in regaining health, obtain as much information as possible from doctors and others, and make sure you are seeing a physician who is knowledgeable about the disease and willing to consult with those who are more knowledgeable..."

Treatment

Standard treatment for NTM infections may include long-term antibiotic therapy and/or surgery. In cases where the infection is confined to one lobe of the lung it may benefit the patient to have the affected lobe removed.

Specialists often recommend a combination of surgery and long-term antibiotic therapy.

These treatments depend on the unique conditions of the patient and the decisions of both patient and physician.

Susceptibility testing should be conducted before antibiotic treatment can begin.

Susceptibility Testing

In the previous chapter you learned about the sputum culture. After the mycobacteria are cultured from the sputum sample, susceptibility testing is done to discover which drugs are most effective for treating the patient.

Multiple Drug Therapy

NTM, and MAC in particular, have a strong natural resistance to antimycobacterial drugs when used independently; as many as 2-6 antibiotics may be recommended by your doctor at one time. Some of the typically administered drugs used to treat NTM and MAC may include:

- Amikacin (Amikin)
- Azithromycin (Zithromax)
- Cefoxitin (or Mefoxin)
- Ciprofloxacin (Cipro)
- Clarithromycin (Biaxin)
- Clofazimine (Lamprene)

Chapter 6 - How is NTM Treated?

- Doxycycline (Vibramycin)
- Ethambutol (Myambutol)
- Imipenem (Primaxin)
- Isoniazid
- Levofloxacin (Levaquin)
- Linezolid
- Moxifloxacin (Avelox)
- Mycobutin (Rifabutin)
- Rifampin (Rifadin, Rifampicin, Rimactane)
- Tigecycline (Tygacil)
- Tobramycin (Nebcin)
- Trimethoprim Sulfamewthoxazole
- Streptomycin

Before taking any drug be sure you understand the directions for use, proper dosages, possible side affects, and foods to avoid.

Amikacin

Amikacin (or Amikin) is an aminoglycoside antibiotic used to treat different types of bacterial infections. Amikacin may be administered once or twice a day but must be given intravenously or intramuscularly. Unfortunately, this procedure can be painful. There is no oral form available. Amikacin is most often used for treating severe infections.

Kidney damage and hearing loss are the most important side effects of Amikacin. Because of this potential, blood levels of the drug and markers of kidney function (creatinine) should be monitored.

Tell your doctor if you experience any of these side affects:

- Dizziness
- Ringing in the ears
- Hearing loss
- Skin rash
- Difficulty breathing
- Difficult or painful urination
- Muscle twitching

Azithromycin

Azithromycin (or Zithromax) is used to treat bacterial and mycobacterial infections; it belongs to the group of drugs called macrolide antibiotics.

Take this drug as directed by your physician. You should take this drug (capsules) on an empty stomach (at least one hour before or two hours after a meal). You should not use azithromycin with antacids and be sure your physician knows if you are taking any blood thinning drugs.

While taking Azithromycin for more than one week, doctors recommend that you get a hearing test and balance test every two to four weeks.

Tell your doctor if you experience any of these side affects:

- Rash or hives
- Dizziness
- Hearing problems
- Wheezing or trouble breathing
- Swelling of the face
- Yellow skin or eyes
- Severe vomiting

Cefoxitin

Cefoxitin (or Mefoxin) is an antibiotic. Cefoxitin kills bacteria that cause infection, or stops the growth of bacteria. Cefoxitin treats many kinds of infections including those of the skin, bone, stomach, respiratory tract, blood, sinuses, ears, and urinary tract.

Diarrhea is a common problem caused by antibiotics which usually ends when the antibiotic is discontinued. Sometimes after starting treatment with antibiotics, patients can develop watery and bloody stools (with or without stomach cramps and fever) even as late as two or more months after having taken the last dose of the antibiotic. If this occurs, patients should contact their physician as soon as possible.

Tell your doctor if you experience any of these side affects:

- Difficulty breathing, wheezing
- Dizziness
- Fever or chills, sore throat
- Headache
- Pain or difficulty passing urine
- Pain, swelling and irritation at the injection site
- Redness, blistering, peeling or loosening of the skin, including inside the mouth
- Severe or watery diarrhea
- Skin rash, itching
- Swollen joints
- Unusual weakness or tiredness

Ciprofloxacin

Ciprofloxacin (or Cipro) treats infections caused by bacteria and mycobacteria; it belongs to the class of drugs called the quinolone antibiotics.

Take this drug as directed by your physician. Take this drug with plenty of water and drink several glasses of water every day while you are taking Cipro. It is best to take this drug on an empty stomach (one hour before or two hours after a meal). You may take this drug with crackers or toast if it upsets your stomach.

Tell your doctor if you experience any of these side affects:

- Shortness of breath
- Rash or hives
- Seizures
- Severe diarrhea
- Swelling of the face throat or lips

Clarithromycin

Clarithromycin (or Biaxin) is used to treat bacterial infections; it belongs to a group of drugs know as the macrolides.

Take this drug as directed by your physician. You should take these tablets on an empty stomach (one hour before or two hours after a meal). However you may take the drug with toast or crackers if it upsets your stomach.

Tell your doctor if you experience any of these side affects:

- Confusion
- Hallucinations
- Depression
- Nightmares
- Trouble sleeping

Clofazimine

Clofazimine is used to treat bacterial and mycobacterial infections.

Take this drug as directed by your physician. This drug should be taken with food or milk.

Tell your doctor if you experience any of these side affects:

- Dizziness or Drowsiness
- Bloody, black or tarry stool
- Burning abdominal or stomach pain
- Mental depression
- Yellow eyes or skin (most importantly bronzing of skin)

Doxycycline

Doxycycline is a member of the tetracycline antibiotics group and is commonly used to treat a variety of infections. Doxycycline is a semi-synthetic tetracycline invented and clinically developed in the early 1960s and marketed under the brand name Vibramycin.

It should be taken with a full glass of water and patients should be upright for at least 30 minutes after administration to prevent irritation of the esophagus and stomach. Also, there is a slim risk of liver damage during prolonged use of the drug. It is also recommended that it be taken with a small meal of a non-dairy nature if upset stomach, nausea, or fatigue occurs.

Tell your doctor if you experience any of these side affects:

- Blurred vision
- Dizziness
- Severe headache
- Fever, chills, body aches
- Skin rash

- Urinating less than usual or not at all
- Dark colored urine
- Nausea and vomiting
- Fast heart rate
- Loss of appetite
- Jaundice (yellowing of the skin or eyes)
- Easy bruising or bleeding

Ethambutol

Ethambutol (or Myambutol) is an antibacterial used to treat tuberculosis (TB).

Take this drug as directed by your physician. This drug may be taken with food if it upsets your stomach. Be sure to have regular eye exams while taking this drug even if you do not notice any changes in your vision.

Tell your doctor if you experience any of these side affects:

- Blurred vision
- Confusion
- Fever
- Inability to see the colors red and green
- Numbness or tingling of the extremities
- Sudden changes in vision
- Skin rash or itching
- Vomiting

Imipenem

Imipenem (or Primaxin) is an antibiotic that fights serious infections caused by bacteria. Cilastatin helps Imipenem work more effectively by preventing the breakdown of the antibiotic in the kidneys. Imipenem and Cilastatin are used to treat severe infections of the lower respiratory tract, skin, stomach, female reproductive organs, and other body systems.

Tell your doctor if you experience any of these side affects:

- Difficulty breathing
- Hives or rash
- Swelling of your face, lips, tongue or throat
- Fast or pounding heartbeat
- Diarrhea that is watery or bloody
- Confusion, tremors, hallucinations, seizure (convulsions)
- Feeling light-headed, fainting
- Fever, chills, body aches, flu symptoms
- Nausea, stomach pain, low fever, loss of appetite, dark urine, clay-colored stools, jaundice (yellowing of the skin or eyes)
- Sore throat, headache, peeling or red skin

Isoniazid

Isoniazid, is used to treat tuberculosis (TB).

Take this drug as directed by your physician. This drug may be taken with food if it upsets your stomach. Take tablets one hour before or two hours after a meal. Isoniazid may be taken with food to avoid upset stomach. Do NOT drink alcohol while taking isoniazid. Be sure your physician knows if you are taking blood thinners, birth control pills, Dilantin or antabuse. If you take antacids wait at least one hour after taking them before taking your Isoniazid dose. Foods such as cheese or fish may cause headache, flushing, pounding heartbeat, sweating, dizziness, chills or diarrhea.

Tell your doctor if you experience any of these side affects:

- Blurred vision or eye pain
- Numbness and/or tingling of extremities
- Yellow skin or eyes
- Dark or amber colored urine
- Severe stomach pain
- Nausea or vomiting
- Weakness
- Fever

Levofloxacin

Levofloxacin (or Levaquin) treats infections caused by bacteria and mycobacteria. It belongs to a group of drugs called the quinolone antibiotics.

Take this drug as directed by your physician. You should take these tablets on an empty stomach (one hour before or two hours after a meal). However you may take the drug with toast or crackers if it upsets your stomach. Do NOT take this medication with large amounts or calcium, such as milk, yogurt or cheese. Do not use antacids with Levaquin. Be sure your doctor is aware if you are taking insulin or other medications to treat diabetes. You may have high or low blood sugar more often while using this drug. Tell your doctor if you are using blood thinners.

Tell your doctor if you experience any of these side affects:

- Rash, hives or peeling red skin
- Swelling of the face, throat or lips
- Wheezing or trouble breathing
- Chest tightness or fast heartbeat
- Seizures, tremors

Chapter 6 - How is NTM Treated?

- Severe diarrhea
- Pain above the heel of your foot
- Pain in the shoulder

Linezolid

Linezolid is a synthetic antibiotic belonging to a new class of antimicrobials called the oxazolidinones. Linezolid disrupts bacterial growth by inhibiting the initiation process of protein synthesis--a mechanism of action that is unique to this class of drugs. It is well absorbed with high bioavailability.

Eating tyramine while you are taking linezolid can raise your blood pressure to dangerous levels. Avoid foods that have a high level of tyramine such as:

- Aged cheeses or meats
- Pickled or fermented meats
- Sauerkraut
- Soy sauce
- Tap beer (alcoholic or non alchololic)
- Red wine
- Any meat or cheese or other protein-based food that has been improperly stored

Tell your doctor if you experience any of these side affects:

- Difficulty breathing
- Blurred vision or trouble seeing colors
- Pale skin, easy bruising or bleeding
- Fever, chills, body aches, flu symptoms
- Diarrhea that is watery or bloody

- Numbness, burning, pain, or tingly feeling in your hands or feet
- Seizure (convulsions)
- Muscle pain, numb or cold feeling in your arms/legs
- Nausea with vomiting
- Fast or irregular heartbeat
- Unusual weakness

Moxifloxacin

Moxifloxacin (or Avilox) is an antibiotic prescribed to treat sinus and lung infections. It kills bacteria that can cause sinusitis, pneumonia, and secondary infections in chronic bronchitis. It also fights skin infections caused by staph or strep.

Moxifloxacin is a member of the quinolone family of antibiotics. Like all antibiotics, Moxifloxacin works only against bacteria.

Tell your doctor if you experience any of these side affects:

- Diarrhea
- Dizziness
- Skin rash or hives
- Tingling
- Fast or irregular heartbeat
- Shortness of breath
- Swelling of the face or throat
- Difficulty swallowing

Mycobutin

Mycobutin (or Rifabutin) is antibacterial and mycobacterial drug.

Take this drug as directed by your physician. Rifabutin may be taken on an empty stomach (either one hour before or two hours after a meal). However, if this medicine upsets your stomach, you may want to take it with food. This drug will discolor normal bodily secretions like tears and urine.

Tell your doctor if you experience any of these side affects:

- Diarrhea
- Fever
- Heartburn or indigestion
- Loss of appetite
- Nausea
- Skin itching and/or rash

Rifampin

Rifampin (or Rifadin, Rifampicin, Rimactane) treats tuberculosis and other infections.

Take this drug as directed by your physician. Rifampin should be taken on an empty stomach (one hour before or two hours after a meal). It is important to take Rifampin on a regular schedule. Do not drink alcohol while taking this medicine. Birth control pills may not work while you are taking Rifampin.

Tell your doctor if you experience any of these side affects:

- Nausea and vomiting
- Yellowing skin or eyes
- Fever
- Blurred vision or eye pain
- Bloody or very dark urine
- Unusual bleeding or bruising

Tigecycline

Tigecycline is an glycylcycline antibiotic. Tigecycline injection solution is for infusion into a vein. Tigecycline is usually first given in a hospital or clinic for severe infections. If you are to give yourself tigecycline by infusion at home, follow the directions on the prescription label. Finish the full course prescribed by your prescriber or health care professional even if you think your condition is better. Do not stop using except on your prescriber's advice. Make sure you understand how to store and give yourself tigecycline. Ask your prescriber or health care professional if you have any questions.

Tell your doctor if you experience any of these side affects:

- Difficulty breathing
- Fever
- Increased sensitivity to light
- Irregular heart beat
- Redness, blistering, peeling of the skin
- Severe diarrhea
- Skin rash, itching
- Unusual weakness or fatigue
- Severe nausea or vomiting
- Swelling of the hands or feet
- Yellowing of the eyes or skin

Tobramycin

Tobramycin sulfate, is an antibiotic used to treat a wide variety of serious bacterial infections, including respiratory infections, skin infections, urinary tract infections and infections of the blood, abdomen and bones. This medication must be given by injection since it is poorly absorbed if taken by mouth.

Kidney damage, nerve damagae and hearing loss are the most important side effects of Tobramycin. Because of this potential, blood levels of the drug and markers of kidney function (creatinine) should be monitored.

Tell your doctor if you experience any of these side affects:

- Dizziness
- Ringing in the ears
- Hearing loss
- Skin rash
- Difficulty breathing
- Difficult or painful urination
- Unusual amount of urine
- Numbness
- Muscle twitching
- Seizures

Trimethoprim Sulfamethoxazole

Trimethoprim Sulfamewthoxazole (Bactrim or Septra) is combination of two antibiotics used to treat a wide variety of bacterial infections, for exampple: middle ear, urinary, respiratory and intestinall infections. It is also used to prevent and treat a specific type of pneumonia (pnemocystis). Take this medication by mouth with a full glass of water.

Some people are allergic to TMP/SMX. Be sure to tell your health care provider if you are allergic to sulfa drugs or antibiotics. People who are anemic should not use TMP/SMX. Taking TMP/SMX during pregnancy may increase the risk of birth defects. Women who are pregnant or breastfeeding should avoid taking it if possible. Also let your health care provider know if you have liver disease, kidney disease, or a shortage of the enzyme glucose-6-phosphate dehydrogenase (G6PD).

If stomach upset occurs, take with food or milk. Drink plenty of fluids while taking this medication to prevent unlikely kidney stones from forming, unless your doctor advises you otherwise.

Tell your doctor if you experience any of these side affects:

- Muscle weakness
- Mental/mood changes
- New lump/growth in the neck (goiter)
- Blood in the urine, dark urine
- Change in the amount of urine
- Confusion
- Persistent headache
- Neck stiffness
- Seizures
- Skin rash, itching, swelling, blisters
- Persistent sore throat
- Paleness
- Joint pain/aches
- Persistent cough
- Trouble breathing
- Easy bleeding/bruising
- Yellowing eyes or skin
- Persistent nausea/vomiting
- Unusual fatigue

Streptomycin

Streptomycin is used for treating tuberculosis (TB) and infections caused by certain bacteria.

Streptomycin is an aminoglycoside. It works by killing sensitive bacteria by stopping the production of essential proteins needed by the bacteria to survive.

Lab tests, including kidney function and complete blood cell counts, may be performed to monitor your progress or to check for side effects. Be sure to keep all doctor and lab appointments.

Tell your doctor if you experience any of these side affects:

- Dizziness, lightheadedness, loss of balance
- Difficulty breathing
- Tightness in the chest
- Swelling of the mouth, face, lips or tongue
- Decreased urination
- Headache
- Hearing loss
- Muscle weakness
- Nausea or vomiting
- Numbness or tingling
- Ringing or roaring in the ears
- Skin rash, itching or hives
- Vaginal irritation or discharge

Oral Medication

Oral medication is part of the treatment picture. In some cases, often when a specific mycobacteria is not susceptible to medication normally taken by mouth, intravenous (IV) medication is indicated.

Intravenous Medication

IV medicines are those that are administered into the vein. The IV infusion method is more complex than simply swallowing a few capsules but vitally important for those infected with the more drug resistant forms of mycobateria.

Inhaled Medication

Inhaled drugs may be prescribed. These drugs are normally administered by inhaler or nebulizer.

An inhaler usually contains premeasured amounts of medication that is inhaled to ease breathing or medicate the lungs. A nebulizer is a device used to reduce liquid to an extremely fine cloud, especially for delivering medication to the deep part of the respiratory tract.

Information and video on how to use a nebulizer can be found at:

http://www.njhealth.org... Type "nebulizer" in the search box.

Other Things You Can Do

Other things you can do to help improve your rate of recovery and health include:

- Nasal Wash
- Airway Clearance
- Exercise
- Proper Diet
- Adequate Sleep

Nasal Wash

Many people with NTM and MAC also have nasal and sinus symptoms. The nasal passages are lined with a thin layer of mucus that traps and eliminates dust, dirt, pollen and other airborne impurities. Some believe that mycobacteria become trapped in the mucus and may find their way into the lungs where they have a perfect medium to grow and flourish.

Drainage from the nose and sinuses can aggravate any condition, especially at night. A salt-water nasal wash:

- Cleans mucus from the nose and alleviates post nasal drip
- Clears allergens and irritants from the nose
- Decreases swelling in the nose. Some devices that aid in nasal irrigation are:
    - NeilMed Sinus Rinse kit
    - Neti Pot

NeilMed Sinus Rinse Kit
The NeilMed Sinus Rinse Kit provides a plastic easy squeeze bottle, premeasured saline packets and complete instructions for use.

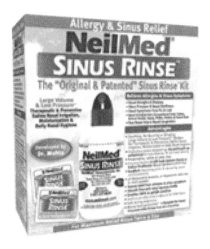

The plastic bottle is filled with eight ounces of room temperature, distilled water and the contents of the Sinus Rinse packet, which is pH balanced, and contains a preservative free mixture of sodium chloride and sodium bicarbonate. The procedure for use follows:

1. Secure the cap and tube to the bottle and shake to dissolve the mixture.

2. Next, with the mouth open and the cap pressed snugly against the nasal opening, gently squeeze the bottle until the solution drains from the opposite nostril.

3. Repeat on the other nasal passage. Two to four ounces are used for each rinse. It is recommended that this procedure be performed once a day, only in the morning.

4. The bottle must be thoroughly cleaned with alcohol and left to drain.

It is best to speak with your physician about this procedure and always follow the manufacturer's directions. For more information about the Neil Med Sinus Rinse Kit and Sinus Rinse Mixture Packets contact NeilMed products at:

- 877-477-8633
- http://www.neilmed.com

Chapter 6 - How is NTM Treated?

Neti Pot

Another nasal wash option is the Neti Pot. The Neti Pot has been used for decades to ensure free airflow through both nostrils

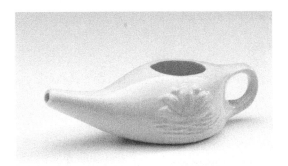

The Neti Pot is shaped like an Alladin's Lamp; it is a small ceramic pot with a small spout that fits into the nostril and the liquid mixture is gently poured into the nasal passage. Some users prefer this Neti method because there is no pressure to affect the ears. Always perform your nasal wash before noon. This will allow any residual water to drain during the remainder of the day.

1. First, mix one Neilmed Sinus Rinse packet in eight ounces of distilled water at room temperature.

2. Pour four ounces of the mixture into the Neti Pot.

3. Start with the right nostril so there is no confusion about which nostril you rinsed and which one remains to be rinsed.

4. Over a sink or basin, insert the spout so it forms a seal and raise the pot so the solution flows into the nasal passage and out the opposite nostril. Open mouth.

5. When the pot is empty, exhale to expel any remaining solution.

6. Refill the Neti Pot and repeat on the opposite side.

7. Drain any remaining saline by bending forward far enough so that the top of the head is pointing toward the floor. Let your arms and head hang freely for a few seconds. All water will drain.

Remember, the nasal wash is not a substitute for medical treatment. It is best to speak with your physician about this procedure and always follow the manufacturer's directions. For more information about the Neti Pot see the internet for many options or contact Himalayan Institute at:

- 1-800-822-4547

- http://www.himalayaninstitute.org/Netipot/NetiPotGateway.aspx

Airway Clearance

Airway clearance is the clearance of mucus from the airways in your lungs. For those with NTM and/or MAC, airway clearance is very important. If bronchiectasis is present, it is often difficult or impossible to cough. As a result, infected mucus stays in the lungs and can decrease lung function. Airway clearance will help remove infected mucus and help preserve lung function over the long term. Vigorous exercise is also very helpful in clearing mucus.

Two common tools for airway clearance include:

- Acapella Choice
- Flutter® Valve

Acapella Choice

The Acapella Choice is intended for use by patients with lung disease and associated airway clearance problems (bronchiectasis).

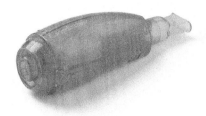

Regular use of the device can significantly improve the clearance of mucus in the lungs. It is easy to use and facilitates opening of airways. The device can be used in any position; patients are free to sit, stand, or recline. You will need a prescription from your physician to purchase an acapells. Remember to clean the acapella daily and disinfect it weekly. Do NOT inhale through the acapella as this may cause reinfection. The product has a life span of approximately one year and costs about $69.95.

For correct instructions on how to use an acapella, NTM patients should go to the National Jewish Health web site and type Acapella-Choice in the search box:

http://www.nationaljewishhealth.org/

You may watch a video about the Acapella Choice on the Smiths Medical web site at:

http://www.smiths-medical.com/education-resources/videos/respiratory/index.html

You may purchase the Acabella with a prescription at:

http://www.activeforever.com

Flutter® Valve

Much like the Acapella device, the Flutter® Valve is a hand held device that helps a patient expel respiratory secretions. It is shaped somewhat like a pipe.

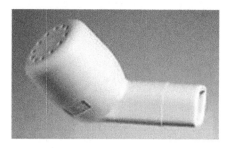

When the patient exhales through the Flutter®, the result is a vibrating of the airway walls, which loosens secretions. The positioning or angle of the Flutter® will determine the vibration level. Special cough maneuvers can be used to remove the secretions.

You will need a prescription from your physician to purchase this item. The Flutter® Valve can be ordered for $63.82 from Care Express in Cary Illinois. Purchase the Flutter® Valve (item number SCA.930) at:

http://www.careexpress.com/ or 1-800-339-3880.

Huff Coughing

Huff coughing is a controlled coughing technique used primarily by patients suffering from a lung disease, such as NTM, bronchiectasis or cystic fibrosis. Since forceful coughing can cause airways in patients with a lung disease to collapse, huffing is not as forceful as a cough but can work better and be less tiring. By using the huff coughing technique, patients can effectively clear the airways of mucus that obstructs the airways and causes respiratory distress.

1. First expel all air in your lungs and airways. Begin by slowing down your breathing. Take slow gentle breaths, ending with one slow exhalation lasting three to four seconds.

2. Inhale slowly using your diaphragm. This is called diaphragmatic breathing or "breathing with your belly". This inhalation should be a slow comfortable breath; do not over inflate your lungs.

3. Slowly inhale, hold it for 3 seconds. This is done to control your breathing and prepare for an effective huff cough.

4. Tilt your chin up slightly and use your stomach muscles to make a series of three rapid exhalations with the airway open, making a "ha, ha, ha" sound. This helps to open the epiglottis in your throat and better allow the expulsion of the mucus in your airways.

5. Gain control of your breathing again by taking a few slow breaths.

6. Repeat the huff coughing technique until the mucus has reached the back of your throat, then cough to expel it. Reclining to cough often helps.

Exercise

Exercise affects NTM patients in many positive ways. It improves lung function, reduces fatigue, improves blance, and strengthens muscles and bones. Exercise also reduces stress and improves circulation. Overall, exercise positively affects every system in the body, including the immune system, the lymphatic system and respiratory system. To regain health, it is important to exercise regularly.

Simple exercise programs can greatly improve your quality of life. Talk to your doctor about an exercise program tailored to your capability. Physical rehabilitation and therapy may be an option for you. If your condition requires no restrictions, a personal trainer may be able to help you build strength and confidence to become fit and healthy.

> **Carole from Massachusetts**
>
> "I walk 50 minutes a day and I take Ballroom Dancing lessons. I do everything I did before I got sick. I will control it. I refuse to let it control me."

Proper Diet

Some nutritional management is important with infectious disease. While your body is being challenged by and treated for illness it is important to be sure you are getting all the vitamins and minerals necessary for good health. A vitamin and mineral product that contains all the necessary vitamins and minerals needed for your age group should be taken daily.

The need for protein is increased when NTM is present.

Increased Protein

Protein is the major component of muscles, bones, enzymes, hormones and antibodies needed to fight infection. Healthy adult men should consume approximately 56 grams of protein per day; adult women about 45 grams per day.

When an infectious disease like NTM is present the need for protein is greater. During illness, antibiotic therapy and recovery, men should consume approximately 90 grams of protein per day; adult women about 80 grams per day.

The easiest method to calculate needed protien for NTM patients in grams for your body weight is to divide by 2. For example, 122 pounds $\div 2 = 61$ grams of protein.

If maintaining your weight is a problem, speak with your physician about ways you might improve nutrition. You may also elect to visit a nutritionist.

Tips for Adding More Protein to Your Diet

Include more protein with each meal by:

- Adding cottage cheese to meals
- Replacing milk with half and half
- Adding grated cheese to soups, salads, vegetables and sauces
- Adding cheese and or meat to sandwiches
- Using more peanut butter
- Adding tuna to salads, sandwiches, or sauces
- Including eggs in dishes and meals
- Adding protein drinks to your meals
- Snacking on protein bars between meals

Adequate Sleep

Sleep is an important aid to the healing process. At least eight hours of sleep every night is necessary to regain and maintain health. Be sure to allow for eight hours of sleep every night. Improve the quality of your sleep by letting yourself wind down and relax before retiring. Do something that helps you to sleep, like reading or taking a warm bath.

Remember that exercising during the day will usually ensure that you sleep at night.

Summary

As a result of reading this chapter, you are now able to:

- Identify some of the major antibiotics used in treatment of NTM such as:
    - Amikacin
    - Azithromycin
    - Cipro
    - Clarithromycin
    - Ethambutol
    - Isoniazid
    - Levofloxacin
    - Moxifloxacin
    - Mycobutin
    - Rifampin

- Discuss other components of the standard protocol and how they benefit the patient; for instance:
    - Nasal Wash
    - Airway Clearance
    - Exercise
    - Proper Diet
    - Adequate Sleep

Chapter 7   Regaining and Maintaining Health

Overview

This chapter will describe important measures for regaining and maintaining health. In addition, you will learn about some supplemental measures that may accelerate your recovery and protect you from reinfection.

As a result of reading this chapter you will be able to:

- Identify important measures for regaining and maintaining health

- Discuss supplemental measures that may accelerate your recovery

---

Debbie Breslawsky *of Weston, Connecticut, is 62 years old. She experienced a chronic cough for 30 years; in 2000 she was diagnosed with pneumonia. Her pulmonologist sent her sputum samples to National Jewish Health for specialized examination. Debbie was diagnosed and treated for NTM. She flip flops between positive and negative sputum cultures. M. abscessus, and M. chelonae have been cultured and treated in Debbie's medical history.*

Debbie stays fit by walking, skiing, and practicing Yoga. She returns to National Jewish Health twice yearly and stays current with what's happening in the diagnosis and treatment of NTM.

Today, Debbie is an NTM activist; she facilitates an NTM support group, serves as a National Trustee of National Jewish Health and attends the annual efforts to lobby congress for more research into the causes and cures for NTM.

Important Measures

Important measures that, when adhered to conscientiously, will assist the NTM patient in regaining and maintaining health include:

- Use of prescribed medications
- Regular exercise
- Increased protein intake
- Extra fluid intake
- Daily nasal washes
- Daily airway clearance
- Using facemasks
- Shower protection

Use of Prescribed Medications

NTM patients are most commonly treated with multiple medications. Because the mycobacteria can mutate and become resistant to drugs, it is extremely important to take the prescribed medications in the correct amounts on a daily basis, for the prescribed length of time. It is important NOT to stop taking the medication. Often patients begin to feel much better and are tempted to stop the medication. This would NOT be beneficial. Your physician will let you know when the mycobacteria have been controlled for a long enough period that you may go off the medication.

Medications may be prescribed in the form of:

- Oral medication
- Intravenous medication
- Inhaled medication

To regain and maintain health take all prescribed medication/s religiously.

Regular Exercise

Many people with NTM report that exercise helps improve strength and stamina. The heavy breathing associated with daily exercise helps to clear the lungs of mucus and helps keep the respiratory, circulatory and immune systems healthy.

Exercise helps to improve circulation, which brings new, oxygenated blood to the lungs as well as all parts of the body.

To regain and maintain health, exercise daily.

> **Debbie from Connecticut**
>
> "I exercise whenever possible. I walk, ski and practice yoga... which has helped. For the most part, I feel terrific. I have a great deal of energy for most of the day."

Increased Protein Intake

The daily requirement of calories and protein for healthy adults is:

- Men – 2700 calories with 56 grams of protein
- Women – 2000 calories with 45 grams of protein

When infectious disease like NTM is present, the need for protein is greater. During illness, antibiotic therapy and recovery more protein is needed.

The formula for protein requirements is about 1 gram of protein per kilogram of body weight. Convert pounds to kilograms by dividing body weight by 2, for example: 124 pounds ÷ 2 = 62 kilograms. Next multiply 62 x 1 = 62 grams. So, a 124 pound person would require 62 grams of protein daily if infectious disease like NTM is present.

If maintaining your weight is a problem speak with your physician about ways in which you might improve nutrition. You may also see a nutritionist.

Protein is the major component of muscles, bones, enzymes, hormones and antibodies needed to fight infection. Keep in mind that protein is needed to oppose NTM and regain health. Include more protein with each meal by:

- Adding cottage cheese to meals
- Replacing milk with Half and Half
- Adding grated cheese to soups, salads, vegetables and sauces
- Adding cheese and meat to sandwiches
- Using more peanut butter
- Adding tuna to salads, sandwiches or sauces
- Including eggs in dishes and meals
- Adding protein drinks to your meals
- Snacking on protein bars between meals

Extra Fluid Intake

NTM patients benefit from drinking at least 10 eight-ounce glasses of water every day. Adequate fluid intake helps decrease the thickness of mucus which makes it easier to loosen and cough up secretions. Some drinks, like caffeinated beverages (coffee, tea and cola) and alcohol have a diuretic effect on the body and actually dehydrate the system. These drinks should be avoided. The rule of thumb for people over 100 pounds is to consume a total fluid intake of half the body weight in ounces. For example, a 180-pound person should consume 90 ounces of water daily. Drink water and juice whenever possible.

Extra fluid intake also helps the kidneys and liver process and remove by-products of the medications.

Daily Nasal Washes

The nasal wash, described earlier, is easy to do and has a refreshing effect. Nasal rinsing results in a clean fresh sensation that allows free breathing, diminishes nasal drainage and may totally eliminate postnasal drip.

Daily Airway Clearance

Airway clearance with either the Flutter® Valve or Acapella helps loosen and eliminate mucus that would otherwise be almost impossible to expectorate. Your physician may prescribe another method if airway clearance is not accomplished with either of these methods.

Regardless of which method is chosen or preferred, airway clearance is necessary to regain and maintain health for the NTM patient.

Using Facemasks

The Food and Drug Administration (FDA) and Center for Disease Control (CDC) define two types of respiratory safety masks - facemasks and respirators.

A **facemask** is a loose-fitting, disposable device that creates a physical barrier between your mouth and nose and potential contaminants in the immediate environment. If worn properly, a facemask is meant to help block large-particle droplets, splashes, sprays or splatter that may contain germs (viruses and bacteria) from reaching your mouth and nose. Facemasks also reduce exposure of your saliva and respiratory secretions to others. While a facemask may be effective in blocking splashes and large-particle droplets, a facemask, by design, does not filter or block very small particles in the air that may be transmitted by coughs, sneezes or certain medical procedures. Facemasks do not provide complete protection from germs and other contaminants because of the loose fit between the surface of the facemask and your face. Facemasks are not intended to be used more than once.

A **respirator** is a protective device designed to achieve a very close facial fit and very efficient filtration of airborne particles. Non-disposable and disposable respirators are available. A 'N95' designation means that when subjected to careful testing, and if properly fitted, the respirator blocks at least 95% of very small test particles. To work as expected, a N95 respirator requires a proper fit to your face. Fit testing is recommended for optimal effectiveness. N95 respirators are not designed for children or people with facial hair as a proper fit cannot be achieved and the respirator may not provide full protection. Disposable respirators are not intended to be used more than once.

A few minutes of research on the Internet will provide you substantial information about facemasks and respirators. Visit the CDC web site at http://www.cdc.gov and search on the keywords "masks" and "respirators". Visit http://www.youtube.com for demonstrations about how to fit facemasks and respirators properly.

Some NTM patients believe that they benefit from the added protection that a facemask provides while performing certain household tasks where dust or bacteria (aerosolized or otherwise) might be inhaled. Activities may include:

- Traveling
- Gardening
- Vacuuming
- Sweeping, dusting or sanding

Traveling
Crowded planes, trains and buses are sources of all types of bacteria and virus contagion. Many NTM patients opt to use facemask protection while traveling. While facemasks provide barrier protection against droplet and contact transmission of virus, they do not protect against inhalation of very small airborne particles. Disposable facemasks should be discarded after use.

Gardening
Gardening can pose a problem for the NTM patient because mycobacteria are found in soil and water. Facemasks can protect patients from breathing large amounts of soil and dust while gardening. While disposable facemasks offer some protection, a properly fitted respirator may offer greater protection.

Vacuuming

Many NTM patients opt to use a facemask while using any dust creating equipment. The vacuum cleaner is notorious for spewing fine particles of dust and debris into the air. Soil, chemicals, fertilizers, and other types of filth can be tracked into the home when outdoor shoes are worn indoors. The vacuum cleaner then hurls the contaminants into the air so that the compromised patient could inhale the dust.

Sweeping, Dusting or Sanding

Activities that can raise dust of dirt into the air can be dangerous for a person with NTM. Patients should be thoughtful about exposure to such environmental conditions. NTM patients with bronchiectasis should be especially careful.

Shower Protection

While many physicians instruct their NTM patients to avoid showers, waterfalls, steam and hot tubs, and it seems prudent to do so, some NTM patients shower with caution. If you can't give up showering, physicians suggest:

- Increasing the hot water temperature
- Installing metal showerheads
- Using a showerhead filter
- Using exhaust fans
- Increasing air circulation
- Decreasing shower time

Increasing the Hot Water Temperature

Most hot water tanks are set at 120 °F. In the article "The Case for Hot Water" which appeared in ScienceNews magazine in 2008, Janet Raloff states: that the Department of Energy (DOE) notes that, "Although some manufacturers set water heater thermostats at 140 °F, most households usually only require them set at 120 °F." What DOE and other energy-conservation sites don't point out is that 140 °F will kill a number of potentially lethal waterborne organisms, like the ones responsible for Legionnaire's disease and NTM, short for nontuberculous mycobacterial infections. In contrast, 120 °F provides a nurturing environment for such toxic microbes. [10]

Many NTM patients have raised the temperature on their household hot water tanks to at least 122 °F in an attempt to decrease the chance of becoming re-infected by mycobacteria or other organisms.

Installing Metal Showerheads

In September 2009, in Nicholas Wade's article in The New York Times, "Bathing but Not Alone" he explains that a group of microbiologists headed by Norman R. Pace of the University of Colorado, as part of a project to measure microbes in the indoor human environment, looked at shower water, in part because in showers bacteria are incorporated into fine droplets that can be breathed deep into the lungs.[11]

Mycobacterium avium tends to be a particular problem in municipal water supplies, Dr. Pace said. The reason is that cities treat their water with chlorine, a poison that kills most bacteria but gives avium a selective advantage. [12]

The bacteria get into shower heads from the water and build up there, so the dose is highest when the shower is first turned on. Running the water for 30 seconds before stepping in would mean fewer bacteria in one's face, Dr. Pace observed. Also, the bacteria seem to find metal shower heads a less hospitable niche than plastic ones.[13]

Today, many NTM patients have replaced their existing plastic shower heads with safer metal shower heads.

Using a Showerhead Filter

Since most NTM patients are hyper aware of bacteria and conditions that can increase exposure to bacteria many opt for shower filtration. Although the size of most mycobacteria is small enough to penetrate most filtration devices some patients utilize shower filters to eliminate chlorine vapors. Many patients that suffer with asthma regard chlorine shower filters the best.

Also, the Pall Corporation offers a shower head that filters many threatening mycobacteria. The filter has a short life span, about 30 days, but they can be purchased in cartons of twelve. For patients who are immune compromised this filtration option might be helpful. Please see the link below for more information.

http://www.pall.com/medical_47285.asp

http://www.webmd.com/lung/copd/news/20090914/bacteria-may-lurk-on-your-showerhead

Using Exhaust Fans
NTM patients are obviously very concerned about the aerosolized water they maybe exposed to while showering. To reduce this exposure many patients have installed exhaust fans in the shower. Exhaust fans should be:

- Located in or near the shower or tub
- Placed opposite the supply air source to ensure that the fresh air is drawn through the room.

Increasing Air Circulation
To avoid re-infection while showering, NTM patients should allow as much air into the shower area as possible. Suggestions include:

- Keeping the bathroom door ajar
- Keeping the shower door/ curtain partially open
- Decreasing Shower Time

Another way to avoid exposure to mycobacteria is to reduce the amount of time spent showering.

NTM patients share other ideas for minimizing the risk of re-infection such as:

- Allow the shower to run a few minutes to blow out any

build up of mycobacteria in the showerhead

- Open the water mixing valve, by placing the selection knob between shower and bath, to allow any trapped water to drain out (after showering)
- Keep the shower area clean and free of mold
- Clean the showerhead inside and out periodically to avoid biofilm build up.

Supplemental Methods

Supplemental methods that may accelerate an NTM patient's recovery include:

- Positive attitude
- Relaxation techniques
- Positive affirmations

These methods have provided many patients with relief as well as a healthy outlook. There have been many cases where people have overcome the odds to regain health and live happy productive lives.

Positive Attitude

Most of us already know that a positive attitude makes a huge difference in our daily lives. Staying positive makes us feel better, look better and even makes us easier to be around. During the last century psychologist Henry James wrote that, "One of the greatest discoveries of my generation, was that human beings can alter their lives by altering their attitudes of mind." Andrew Weil, M. D. tells us "… that positive thinking can enhance health. Pessimism has been linked to a higher risk of dying before age 65, while positive emotions – such as optimism – are associated with lowered production of the stress hormone cortisol, better immune function and reduced risk of chronic diseases."

Relaxation Techniques

There are volumes written about the benefits of relaxation. Relaxation helps us combat stress by helping us overcome stressors in our daily lives. Because our immune systems are strengthened by relaxation, we can more effectively combat disease to heal and regain health. Two very common relaxation techniques are:

- Progressive muscle relaxation
- Controlled breathing

Progressive Muscle Relaxation

Progressive muscle relaxation is easy to do and can be done any time. First sit or lie in a relaxed position, away from distraction, and take three deep breaths. Now close your eyes and starting with your feet, tighten your feet muscles to the count of five and then release your muscles. Repeat this same procedure upwards to the next muscle group - your lower legs - tighten and hold to the count of five and relax. Next, move upward to your knees, upper legs, hips and so on, up to the scalp. By the time you reach your head you will be perfectly relaxed. You may choose to drift off to sleep at this point or you may sit up and enjoy your rejuvenated, relaxed self.

Controlled Breathing

Controlled breathing can also be done almost anywhere, even at work. All you need is a few minutes in a quiet space. Simply sit in a relaxed position and breath in through your nose, hold for the count of four and exhale through you mouth. Repeat this a total of five breaths and you are finished. You'll be surprised at how refreshed you feel.

Incorporate relaxation techniques into your daily routine and you will notice the impact relaxation will have on your stress level, condition, and total outlook.

Positive Affirmations

Positive affirmations are positive statements used to condition your conscious and unconscious mind towards a healthier outcome.

It is thought that the positive affirmations influence certain parts of the brain, which in turn influence the nervous system and different body functions.

Use positive affirmations by creating short, positive statements that describe the improvement and healthy condition you would like to possess. For example:

- I am happy, healthy, and my immune system is strong
- My respiratory system is strong and healthy
- My lungs are healthy and functioning normally
- I exercise daily to improve my health
- My internal organs function perfectly

Read or recite these affirmations several times every day. To create greater impact, visualize the statement as you recite the affirmation. For example, visualize normal healthy lungs, with healthy, pink tissue… inhaling pure perfect oxygen, and exhaling carbon dioxide in a perfect healthy exchange.

It is believed that after you do this for approximately 30 days, the statements become a part of your belief system and begin to affect change in the system.

Summary

As a result of reading this chapter, you are now able to:

- Identify eight important measures for regaining ad maintaining health:
    - Use of prescribed medications
    - Regular exercise
    - Increased protein intake
    - Extra fluid intake
    - Daily nasal washes
    - Daily airway clearance
    - Use of facemasks
    - Shower protection
- Discuss three supplemental measures that may accelerate your recovery:
    - Positive attitude
    - Relaxation exercises
    - Positive affirmations

Handbook Summary

As a result of reading this handbook, you are now able to:

- Define NTM and its other names:
  - MOTT
  - AM

- Discuss some predisposing factors:
  - Chronic lung disease
  - Inorganic dust exposure

- Identify the symptoms of the NTM:
  - Chronic cough
  - Hemotypsis (bloody sputum)
  - Lowgrade fever
  - Nightsweats

- Discuss how NTM is diagnosed:
  - Chest X-Ray
  - CT Scan
  - Bronchoscopy with culture and sensitivity of samples

- Describe treatment for NTM:
  - Long-term antibiotic therapy with multi drug regimen
  - Possible surgery

- Find resources about NTM:
  - National Jewish Memorial and Research Center
  - NTMinfo.com

Tools You Can Use

The tools listed on the following pages are useful for keeping track of protein consumption, recording medication intake and performing exercises and cleanses. Visit http://www.ntmhandbook.com to download free templates for any of these tracking tools.

Protein Tracker

Acquire a Protein Tracker book at your local bookstore and list the foods you eat on a regular basis. Enter the amount of protein in each food, then track the total amount of protein you consume daily. Make adjustments to your daily intake to move toward healthy limits. Copy the blank Protein Tracker template on the following page, or visit http://www.ntmhandbook.com and click on Resources to download a free template.

Protein Tracker Example

Food	Amount	Grams of Protein
Toast	1 slice	2
Eggs	2	14
Bacon	1 strip	2
Roast Beef	3 oz.	21
Mashed Potatoes	1 cup	4
Cheese	½ cup shredded	14
Cottage Cheese	½ cup	14
Peanuts	¼ cup	10
Carnation Instant Breakfast	8 oz. package	15
Balance Bar	1 bar	20

Protein Tracker

Food	Amount	Grams of Protein

Medication Tracker

List the medications you use on a daily basis and keep track of when you take them. Use the chart below as an example.

Copy the blank Medication Tracker on the following page or go to http://www.ntmhandbook.com and click on Resources to download a free template.

Medication Tracker Example

Med	Mon	Tues	Wed	Thurs	Fri	Sat	Sun
Biaxin 750mg PM	✓	✓					
Ethambutol 800mg AM	✓	✓					
	✓	✓					
Centrum 1 daily	✓	✓					

Medication Tracker

Med	Mon	Tues	Wed	Thurs	Fri	Sat	Sun

Exercise Log

Chart daily exercise to track and increase weekly. See the chart below as an example.

Copy the blank Exercise Log on the following page or go to http://www.ntmhandbook.com and click on Resources to download a free template.

Exercise Log Example

Exercise	Mon	Tues	Wed	Thurs	Fri	Sat	Sun
Treadmill	30 min	30 min					
Sit-Ups	30 min	30 min					
Push-Ups	30 min	30 min					

Exercise Log

Exercise	Mon	Tues	Wed	Thurs	Fri	Sat	Sun

Works Referenced

Daley, Charles. "Nontuberclous Mycobacteria, An Emerging Epidemic." Knol, A Unit of Knowledge 28 July 2008. 10 Nov. 2008 <http://knol.google.com/k/charles-daley/nontuberclous-mycobacteria>.

Dieudonne, M. D., Arry. "Atypical Mycobacterial Infection." eMedicine Journal 16 Oct. 2003. 27 Oct. 2003 <http://author.emedicine.com/PED/topic3034.htm>.

Falkingham, JO III. "Nontuberculous Mycobacteria in the Environment." Clinics in Chest Medicine Sept. 2002, Volume 23 Issue 3 Pages 529-694 <http://www.ncbi.nlm.nih.gov/pubmed/12370991>.

Gorman, Christine. "What's in Your Pipes?" Time 1 July 2002. 5 July 2003 <http://www.time.com>.

Holland, M. D., Steven M. "Laboratory of Host Defenses." National Institute of Health. 17 Dec. 1999. National Institute of Allergy and Infectious Disease. 23 Oct. 2003 <http://www.niaid.nih.gov/dir/labs/lhd/holland.htm>.

Huang, M. D., Judy H. "Mycobacterium avium-intracellulare Pulmonary Infection in HIV-Negative Patients Without Preexisting Lung Disease." Chest Journal 1999. 6 Jan. 2004 <http://www.chestjournal.org/cgi/content/full/115/4/1033>.

Iseman, M. D., Michael D. "Nontuberculous Mycobacteria (NTM)." Medical Scientific Update Spring 1998, Volume 15, Number 4 ed. 9 Jan. 2003 <http://library.nationaljewish.org/MSU/15n4MSU_NTM.html>.

Iseman, M. D., Michael D., Marras, M. D., Theodore K. "The Importance of Nontuberculous Mycobacterial Lung Disease. " American Journal of Respiratory and Critical Care Medicine 5 Nov. 2008 <http://ajrccm.atsjournals.org/cgi/content/full/178/10/999>.

Kim, Brian. "New lung disease lurks in hot tubs and indoor pools that create an infectious mist." The Johns-Hopkins News-Letter 6 Apr. 2000 <http://wwwjhu.edu/~04-6-00/Science/2.html>.

Leitman, Fern. "A Patient's Perspective." NTMinfo.com. 5 July 2002 <http://www.ntminfo.com>.

"MAC (Mycobacterium Avium Complex)." <u>New Mexico AIDS InfoNet</u>. 12 Aug. 2004. New Mexico Department of Health. 27 Oct. 2003 <http://www.aidsinfonet.org/articles.php?articleID=514>.

"Nontuberculous Mycobacteria (NTM)." <u>Medfacts</u> 15 July 2004, National ed. 27 Oct. 2003 <http://www.nationaljewish.org/medfacts/nontuberculosis.html>.

"Reports of Nontuberculous Mycobacterial Infections Increasing in Community Settings." <u>TB Notes Newsletter (CDC)</u> 2002, No. 4 ed. 27 Oct. 2003 <http://www.cdc.gov/nchstp/tb/notes/tbn_4_02/upd_Laboratory.htm>.

"Study Finds Nontuberculous Mycobacteria Lung Disease on the Rise in the United States." <u>NIH News</u> 24 Sept. 2009 <www3.niaid.nih.gov/news/newsreleases/2009/NTMLungDisease.htm>.

Glossary

Acapella Device
An airway clearance device that works by vibration of the airways to mucus so that it can be expectorated.

Anatomical Defects
Defects of the normal anatomy/body.

Brochiectasis
A condition that occurs as a result of chronic or repeated infection of the lungs. May result in permanent dilation of airways, which can cause the loss of structural integrity of the bronchial tree.

COPD
Chronic Obstructive Pulmonary Disease. An acronym for disease that involves airway obstruction such as emphysema and or chronic bronchitis.

Emphysema
A chronic obstructive pulmonary disease in which the lungs lose their elasticity making breathing difficult and inefficient.

Expectorate
To cough or spit out mucus or sputum from the lungs.

Flutter Valve
An airway clearance device that works by vibration of the airways to mucus so that it can be expectorated.

MAC
An acronym for Mycobacterium Avium Complex. MAC is the most common cause of infections due to NTM.

Mucus
Thick secretions found in lungs and sinuses.

NTM
An acronym for Nontuberculous Mycobacteria. NTM is a mycobacterial species other than *M. tuberculosis*. Other acronyms used to describe these same mycobacteria are MOTT (Mycobacteria Other Than Tuberculosis) and AM (Atypical

Mycobacteria).

Predisposing Factor or Condition
An activity or condition which increases the susceptibility to a disease. (a factor like cigarette smoking could predispose one to emphysema... a condition like fair skin could predispose one to sunburn).

PICC Line
A PICC line is a thin flexible silicone tube, the tip of which is placed into one of the large veins in the arm (usually near the bend of the elbow) from where it is threaded into the superior vena cava. The initials PICC stand for peripherally inserted central catheter.

PICC lines are normally inserted as an outpatient. Some local anaesthetic cream is applied to the skin which usually ensures the insertion is painless. The procedure takes about 30 to 40 minutes. Once the PICC line is in place it will be taped firmly to the skin with a special transparent dressing to stop it coming out of the vein. A chest x-ray will then be taken to check the position of the line before it is used.

The PICC line can be used for taking blood for blood tests, giving chemotherapy drugs or giving blood transfusions.

Pulmonary
Of or affecting the lungs.

Risk Factor
Something which increases risk or susceptibility (a fatty diet is a *risk factor* for heart disease).

Sputum
Secretion of the lungs.

Unique Physical Characteristics
Those physical characteristics that make us unique (e. g. height, hair color, weight).

Endnotes

1. Iseman, Michael D. (1998, Spring). *Nontuberculous Mycobacteria (NTM)*. Retrieved January 9, 2003, from http://library.nationaljewish.org/MSU/15n4MSU_NTM.html

2. Ibid

3. About Nontuberculous Mycobacteria. National Jewish Medical and Research Center. Retrieved November, 2007 from http://nationaljewish.org/disease-info/diseases/nts-mycobac/about/index.aspx

4. Iseman, Michael D. (1998, Spring). *Nontuberculous Mycobacteria (NTM)*. Retrieved January 9, 2003, from http://library.nationjewish.org/MSU/15n4MSU_NTM.html

5. Holland, Steven M. (1999, December 17). *Laboratory of Host Defenses*. Retrieved October 23, 2003, from http://www.njaid.nin.gov/dir/labs/lhd/holland.htm

6. Ibid

7. *Nontuberculous Mycobacteria (NTM)*. National Jewish Medical and Research Center. Retrieved October 2003, from http://www.nationaljewish.org/medfacts/nontuberculosis.html

8. Ibid

9. Iseman, Michael D. (1998, Spring). *Nontuberculous Mycobacteria (NTM)*. Retrieved January 9, 2003, from http://library.nationaljewish.org/MSU/15n4MSU_NTM.html

10. Raloff, Janet (2008, October 23). *The Case For Very Hot Water*. Retrieved Feb. 3, 2010 from http://www.sciencenews.org/view/generic/id37933

11. Wade, Nicholas (2009 September 15) *Bathing but Not Alone*. Retrieved Feb. 3, 2010 from http://www.nytimes.com/2009/09/15/health/15shower.html

12. Ibid

13. Ibid

Made in the USA
Las Vegas, NV
03 July 2025